10 LESSONS

FOR USING THE POWER OF LOVE
TO SUCCEED IN LIFE

LOVE YOUR LIFE

AND IT WILL LOVE YOU BACK

SOURENA VASSEGHI

ISBN 0-9791369-0-3
Library of Congress Catalog in Publication Data
i. 1- Self Help 2- Success in Life 3- Cerebral Palsy
ii. Vasseghi, Sourena

Published by
Sourena Publishing
www.LoveYourLifeSeminars.com

January 2007 First Edition.
Printed in Korea
Editors: Barbara McNichol, Carol Givner
Book Design: Stuart Silverstein, stuartsilversteindesign

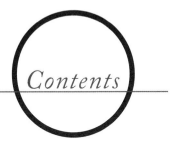

Contents

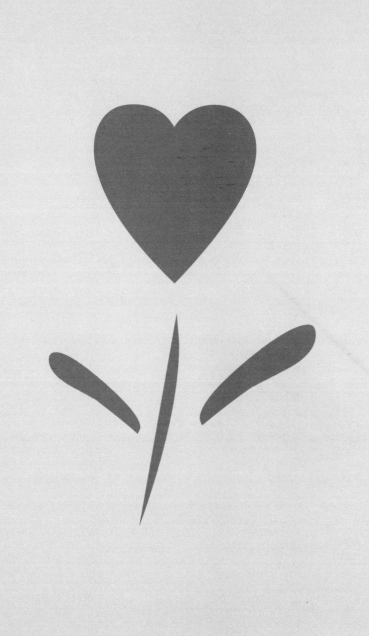

I dedicate this book to my parents, **Zahra and Behzad,**
two people who sacrificed so much for my sister and me.
These amazing people drew the perfect line between
helping me out and letting me find my own path—
I do not know where I would be without them.

Acknowledgments

I would like to thank **Frank Miles,** my wonderful mentor, who helped me take these random thoughts that I had in my brain and organize them. He has also guided me in every step of my speaking business. I don't know what I would do without him.

I would also like to thank:

- **Jay Lavender** who gave me the idea to write this book.
- **Carol Givner** and **Barbara McNichol** who edited this book.
- **Maureen Shampine,** a talent who helped me with many rewrites. I can't wait for her own book!
- **Sierra Feldner-Shaw** who helped me type this book.
- **Stuart Silverstein,** who did the cover design and the layout.
- **Sayyad Chakarian,** who helped me design my website and is a great friend.

Foreword

The word "inspirational" always comes to mind when one is around Sourena Vasseghi for any period of time. Yes, he has a vision for his life, and he has a strong work ethic—his mind is running all the time. He is a total inspiration to everyone with whom he comes in contact as he has the ability to connect the dots of life, when he has not been able to experience it all.

In the classroom at the University of Southern California where I met Sourena in a professor-student relationship, I listened in awe as he would suggest solutions to business issues in the workplace, having NEVER seen the workplace. His innate sense of what is right would prevail, and his fellow students would ask after class how he knew what he was talking about, given that he had not been there.

In fact, their respect for Sourena was so deep that they showed it to him on graduation day:

As the 900 undergraduates walked across the stage to receive their diplomas from the dean, they were excited and scared about what was to come. No one was more so than Sourena, never being able to leave the confines of his wheelchair. I had told all those who were in my classes to "walk slowly—next to your wedding day and the days your children are born, this is the most important day of your life." Most did just that.

Sourena had been waiting in the wings on the stage, and his name was called last. The students rose as one to give him a standing ovation—the only one I had ever seen at graduation. He became so excited that he "popped a wheelie" in his wheelchair, drove out of control across the stage, and almost ran over the dean, whose eyes grew as big as saucers as he set the diploma cover in Sourena's lap.

My last recollection of that day came later that night as I read my students' e-mails from the day. Sourena's merely read, "I screwed up—I went too fast."

Sourena Vasseghi wants to live life fast *and* he wants to enjoy it all. He yearns for the simple things that most people have—the ability to open a wallet and take money out, to kiss a woman and hold her hand, to be one of the group. He is truly an inspiration to me, and always will be. In this book, his ten lessons will be an inspiration to all.

—James G. Ellis,
Professor, University of Southern California

My Life So Far

A t my birth, I was thrown a big curve ball.

Now, I don't believe curve balls or roadblocks are inherently bad. Rather, they are detours inspiring other journeys and providing alternate routes to a destination. Knowing your destination is important, but even more crucial is understanding how to get there when faced with unforeseen roadblocks.

Everyone at some time or another has encountered roadblocks. I've had many and I continue to bump into them every day. But I roll on. Yes, I roll on, knowing that sometimes an answer may be "no," but that does not mean "the end." A "no" simply means getting closer to finding your true path.

> *A "no" simply means getting closer to finding your true path.*

In 1977, the year of my birth, my homeland of Iran brewed with revolution. On October 21st—Friday, the weekly day of rest in Iran—I was about to have a revolution of my own. On that fateful day, I hit my first roadblock, and what an obstacle it would turn out to be! The doctor was not ready for my arrival, so I was deprived of oxygen for ten minutes during the birth process. Those ten minutes would affect and direct my entire life immensely.

Six months after I was born, my parents noticed I wasn't progressing like other children my age. The doctors in Iran had no answers and few suggestions for their obvious concerns, so they wisely began investigating medical facilities in other countries.

When I was two years old, my parents took me to a top medical school at University of California at Los Angeles *(UCLA)*. There, I was officially diagnosed with cerebral palsy *(CP)*, a condition that affects over 750,000 people in the United States alone.. It was caused by the lack of oxygen to my brain during birth. Specifically, CP causes damage to the part of the brain that controls movement and affects motor skills, speech, and sometimes mental capacity. The extent of the damage to my brain, however, was yet unknown.

Consequently, CP has robbed me of muscle control, including the ability to speak clearly. I get around using an electric wheelchair. I need assistance with eating, getting dressed, and using the restroom, among other activities that require muscle movement.

I started my education at a school for the disabled, but after a few years, my teachers recommended that I gradually mainstream into a regular school. In fifth grade, I entered White

Oak Elementary School in Westlake Village, California, still in special education. By the time I was in the seventh grade, I had made my way into all the regular classes, except, of course, for physical education. Which is fine, I never liked dodge ball anyway!

In this new environment, I learned what a normal life could be, especially because everybody at White Oak Elementary treated me as though I belonged in mainstream society without stereotyping me as "the guy in the wheelchair." I enjoyed the popularity I had with my fellow classmates.

Then I went on to high school at Agoura High School in Agoura Hills, CA, where, during summer breaks, my buddies from school included me in whatever they were doing. Through their acceptance, I learned more and more about true friendships. I would love to say we had exciting adventures together, but mostly we just horsed around and goofed off as normal teenage boys do. As naïve as it might sound, I assumed that if I kept rolling along, just as I did with school and summer fun, everything I wanted—the American dream— would fall into my lap: the job, the wife, the house, the white picket fence.

From a young age, I had a fascination with success and business. I grew up watching my dad run three restaurants, two Italian and one Persian, all in the greater Los Angeles area. I was constantly asking my dad questions about them. I always knew I wanted to be a successful businessman.

I had a good upbringing in a loving home. My hardworking parents, Zahra and Behzad, have always provided a comfortable life for my younger sister, Sanaz, and me. I'm able to say that until my early twenties, I had not faced any major roadblocks. I assumed that if I kept plugging away as I always had, all the pieces of my life would simply fall into place.

As time passed, though, a gap grew between my peers and me, marking the starting point of challenges to come: dating, finding a career, and figuring out my place in the world. I have faced these roadblocks one by one and continue to deal with many of them today.

As I entered adulthood, my fascination with achieving success only grew until success became something I felt I *needed.* At that juncture, I let myself fall in love with certain visions and dreams of my success that brought me to where I am today. And although it didn't always seem that life treated me fairly, I discovered that if I loved life enough, it would love me back.

I've written this book as one of the ways I can love life fully—by sharing ten lessons I've learned that I hope will encourage you to love life more fully, too.

I discovered that if I loved life enough, it would love me back.

Introduction to The Ten Lessons

There's a party going on all the time, and it's called **life.**

Imagine walking up to the building where the party's in full swing and hearing music thumping out through the walls. Looking in a window, you can see people dancing with each other, celebrating, laughing, eating their favorite foods. You can't wait; you would do anything in your power to get in.

You have a key to this building where the party is jamming. You try to unlock the door, but it won't open. What do you do? Do you ignore the fact that your key doesn't fit? Do you pretend it does? Do you insist that willpower alone will make it fit if you only keep trying? No, that's crazy! In fact, that will only hinder you from finding the door that truly lets you in. To find that door, it's essential that you embrace not only your talents but your limitations as well. Sure, everybody has limitations. But never look at them as excuses. Instead, they're road maps to keep you on the right path in your life.

The search for finding ways to get into that party can be gut-wrenching. You must believe deep down—with all the love you can muster—that any adversity you may face is only a temporary setback, that you'll get through anything that life throws at you.

It's easy to go through life with your eyes open but without seeing its endless potential, or going through life hearing but not understanding the underlying tones of living. It's also easy to love life when everything is going your way. The true talent is fully loving your life when nothing is going well. You'll experience days when you feel like throwing in the towel, but you have another choice; you can let your love of life carry you through these tough times. Besides, that big party awaits!

---

*The true talent is fully loving your
life when nothing is going well.*

When I was younger, I often feared that no matter how hard I tried, success wouldn't be in the cards for me. Still, I had this passion for life that wouldn't fade away. I tried to convince myself to submit to my disability and accept the destiny that is thrust upon so many disabled people: joblessness, isolation, and a life of insignificance. But a nagging voice kept saying, "Sourena, you have a chance!"

Everything I've learned about success involves integral steps, many of them I'm incapable of taking. Typically, young people are expected to do a myriad of credential-building activities to establish themselves in companies. I was willing but wasn't able to pay my dues—like taking notes easily and running across town on a dime—so I was at a disadvantage. Still, I like learning about the steps taken by famous CEOs such as Donald Trump, Michael Eisner of Disney, Sumner Redstone of Viacom, and Jack Welsh, the former CEO of GE. In fact, as I studied these amazing professionals, I was daunted by many things they did that I could never do. For example, both Trump and Welsh talked about how important golf is for business networking. I think I have the wrong kind of handicap.

While realizing that the conventional ways people achieve success won't work for me, I still knew what I wanted. Slowly, doors that I once thought were shut opened and my life started to love me back because of lessons that I've learned to compensate for my disability. I share ten of these lessons here because I know they can help you achieve success in your life. But first, I have to warn you, don't expect the ordinary! Concepts in this book go against conventional wisdom since I've based all these lessons on love—because I can't think of a better motivator. (When I first conceived of the book, I wanted to compare life to Romeo and Juliet, but then I realized they both died tragically—maybe not the best metaphor for a motivational work!)

Why focus on loving your life as a way to get motivated? Because when you let yourself fully love your life, unspeakable defeats turn into new opportunities!

To fall passionately in love with your life, think like someone who's in that passionate, overwhelming state of being in love. You'll see how they exude these characteristics:

- They have the courage to dream.
- They accept the ones they love exactly the way they are.
- They depend on people for support.
- And, most importantly, they do anything to win the other person's love.

Given that these rewards are waiting for you, then why not fall in love with your life?

This book tells you how I've fallen in love with my own life, despite my physical challenges and the psychological ramifications that have gone with them. Each lesson that follows provides ways to help open doors to this outrageous party called life—and encourages you to live it in a way that will love you back tenfold.

To be passionately in love with your life, think like someone who is deeply in love.

Lesson ①

Dream Your Ideal Life

In the quest for romance and finding the love of your life, it's important to know the attributes of the loved one you seek before setting out to find him or her. You should know the types of people who physically and mentally attract you. You don't simply marry the first passerby you see or even the second. Instead, you sift through the sand to find the perfect sea shell you want to keep. Similarly, to create a successful life, you must have a goal in mind. If you don't know what characteristics you want in your future, you will never reach your goal.

If you don't know what characteristics you want in your future, you will never reach your goal.

One of the most frustrating aspects of my life is that I can't be active all the time. If people aren't available to pick up the slack created by my inability to act, there aren't many things I can do. You see, I have no escape from my disability—a fact that leaves me with a lot of time to reflect on what I want. Very often, people are so busy getting to work, working, coming home, and taking care of errands that they don't have time to reflect on their lives and their dreams. I can tell you right now that if I weren't handicapped, I'd be just like that! I'd be one of those guys eating in the car, talking on the phone, e-mailing people on my Blackberry, and honking at the car in front of me to go faster.

But although I get frustrated when I'm alone with my thoughts, I know it is really a blessing in disguise. My disability has taught me to enjoy the small pleasures of life, such as understanding what true friendship is, making people laugh, and giving back to others.

Today, I'm glad to say I'm living a lifestyle that includes owning my own speaking business, traveling around the world, and enjoying the company of many friends and colleagues. And all the while, I'm in love with life like it's the greatest romance ever!

My disability has taught me to enjoy the small pleasures of life, such as understanding what true friendship is, making people laugh, and giving back to others.

I want to describe a day far in the future, October 21st, 2027. You're probably asking, what's so special about that day? Well, that day will be my 50th birthday. Here is how I imagine it.

I wake up lying beside my wife. I watch her still sleeping and I can't believe how lucky I am to have found her. When she awakens, she leans over and wishes me "Happy Birthday" with a warm, loving kiss. As she gets me ready to face the rest of the day, we reminisce about our years together that have led to that moment.

Later, at breakfast, as my teenage kids tease me about being older than dirt, I look around the house, and I realize that I have achieved many of my aspirations. I own the house that we live in. I'm able to buy my wife the things that give her pleasure. I've taken care of my children's college funds. I feel so proud that I've provided all this for myself and my family.

The rest of the day, I celebrate my 50th birthday with other family members, friends, and colleagues. The best part? That I don't only feel satisfied with my life, but I am still thoroughly in love with it—just as I imagined it over the years.

Every day, I think about success in this form. For me, it means becoming a leader in my industry, having an incredible social and family life, and just being happy to be alive. I've defined my goals specifically enough that I know what I am aiming for, but I also allow for flexibility because I don't know what will pop up. I have no idea what technological changes or medical breakthroughs will occur; I can hardly wait for them!

Most important, I enjoy happiness and success just as I imagined. In my opinion, goals shouldn't be set in stone; they should be dynamic. When goals are dynamic, incalculable opportunities can open up.

For example, if you decide your dream partner must be five-nine, black-haired, brown-eyed and has to like sushi and Steve Martin movies, then you have just narrowed your possibilities. If, however, you describe your future partner as someone who is sensitive and fun to be around, then you'll be more likely to find the special person you're looking for. And if you really want to know the man I've just described, then give me a call!

When goals are dynamic, incalculable possibilities suddenly open up.

I love that dream about how I'll celebrate my 50th birthday so much, there is nothing that I wouldn't do to achieve it. So, I ask, what is your dream? What do you want to see happen? Where do you want to be in the future? Are you on your way to making your own dream real?

At some point or another, you've likely visualized the perfect mate (although there's no such thing as perfect, which, like beauty, is in the eye of the beholder). Don't focus on finding a person who is perfect, but on finding a person who is perfect *for you.*

The same goes for all aspects of your life, job, home, and so on. Identify and fall in love with your dream. Be open to see a myriad of opportunities. And be dedicated enough to your dream to either create opportunities from nothing or take advantage of great ones when they come your way.

Be open to a myriad of opportunities.

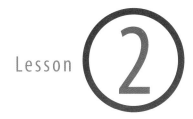

Feel The Fear

In love, you may have the fear of losing a wonderful relationship. This fear keeps you "in line" and helps you appreciate even the less desirable aspects of your mate. To be specific, this fear can inspire a man to go to the ballet or make a woman watch Monday Night Football; it can make you willing to do *anything* to keep what you hold dear.

I am not sure why, but being fearful is frowned upon in our society. Conventional wisdom states that in order to succeed, people must be fearless. But if that's true, why do we put on seat belts when we get into a car? I, for one, have two reasons I feel compelled to put on my seat belt: *(1)* fear of crashing and *(2)* fear of getting a ticket for not wearing a seat belt. People buy life insurance to keep the family safe because of the fear of an unexpected tragedy.

So why not use fear to your advantage in other ways?

I remember two friends in college who were paranoid wrecks the night before taking their exams. Even though they were both honor students, they thought they would "bomb" their tests. The way I saw it, their fear of failure ensured their success because it motivated them to work harder.

I consider fear to be good as long as it motivates you to make a change. Yes, it's easy to become overcome by fear, submit to it, and let it get the better of you. The key to avoid being overcome by fear is to use it to stimulate your passion.

Fear is good as long as it motivates
you to make a change.

Like most adolescents, I started noticing girls when puberty struck in my early teens. I had always wanted to experience a relationship, but I didn't dwell on it. Rather, I convinced myself that if I had patience, a good relationship with a girl would just happen.

The first time I really experienced gut-wrenching fear was around the time I turned twenty. That's when I experienced my first crush—a cute girl from economics class named Molly.

Sure, I envied my classmates going on dates, holding hands with girls in the halls at school, and all that jazz. But because I felt afraid of dealing with the reality of my situation, I ignored any romantic inclinations I had toward Molly for a long time. To state it bluntly, I was so fearful of rejection that I convinced myself inaction was perfectly acceptable. "Everything would magically fall into place," I'd tell myself, ignoring the impracticality of that notion. I believe this is a faulty way of thinking for anyone, much less someone with a disability. I needed to be more proactive, to put myself out there, to pursue this venture diligently.

Now, if you're just hoping what you want will fall into your lap, you're mistaken. By age nineteen, I had come to realize that this wonderful girl wouldn't just fall into my lap, unless, of course, I knocked her over with my wheelchair! So, with some reservation, I decided I would ask Molly out on a date.

At first I was excited at the prospect because, like any normal teenager, I wanted to enjoy dating. The more I thought about asking her, though, the more nervous I became. How would I do it? I decided passing her a letter on the last day of class would be the best way to go about it—for two reasons.

First, I was concerned about being able to communicate verbally. Would she understand me through my speech impediment? I'd always preferred verbal communication despite its difficulties, but in this instance, it seemed too risky. I thought I'd have a better chance of getting a favorable response writing a letter since I could clearly present my thoughts without coming across as feeling nervous. Plus, I wouldn't have to worry about the awkwardness of having to repeat myself when asking her out. After all, it's hard enough to get it out the first time! And I certainly didn't want to emphasize my disability from the get go. I wanted her to see past the wheelchair; to see *me*, Sourena. A letter seemed the best way to accomplish that.

Second, if she said "no" on that last day of class, then I'd never have to see her again, which meant I wouldn't have to feel the embarrassment sitting near her in class every day thereafter!

So I set out to write the perfect letter—until fear started to cloud my thoughts. My biggest question was, "Would she look at me as a man?" And if she did see me as a man and said "yes" to a date, I worried about dealing with a whole new set of fears beyond the usual "where will we go"; "what will we do"; "will she like me?" I would also have to ask "would she be willing to help me in and out of the car?" and "would she be willing to help me eat?" and "would I be able to satisfy her needs?" Now, by saying needs, don't get the wrong idea! I merely mean things like opening a door for her, pulling out her chair, and so on. Would I still be able to make her feel like a woman even though I might not do things a man would normally do?

Not only that, but my mind started to race about the long-term ramifications of her saying "yes" to one date. "Would she go out with me again?" "Would she tire of my special circumstances?" Oh, man! I was playing out the entire relationship before I even wrote one lousy letter!

Despite these seriously daunting questions, I proceeded with the letter writing. Then a good friend convinced me I was being a coward, and that writing the letter wasn't enough. He told me to be confident, forget the letter, and just ask Molly out directly.

This idea terrified me!

Fearful, and faced with the possibility of rejection, still I imagined the dire consequences of not acting at all. Specifically, I was so afraid of ending up alone that I took my friend's advice and forced myself to take action. I was all ready to ask her out the next class I saw her. But the next class came, and as luck would have it, she was absent. Did this girl not realize the effort I had put into my pre-planned declaration of love?!?

So the next time I thought she'd be in class, I got to the end of the hallway, and the elevator to my second story class was out of order. I honestly thought about crawling up the stairs, but I didn't want to get my jeans dirty. Plus, because I was on my knees, I didn't want Molly to think I was proposing to her.

Finally, one fateful day, our class got cancelled and I saw Molly walking toward the library. Let me paint the picture for you. Molly took a seat on a bench and I rolled over to where she was. I, of course, was already seated. The conversation that I had plotted, planned, prayed, and agonized over for six weeks went something like this:

Me: "Will you go out with me? I'm normal."

Now, I know other words came out too, but honestly, I was so nervous, I don't remember them. I was rambling. I took a breath and there hung my request—raw and abrupt.

I waited for her reply.

Molly: "Oh Sourena, I already have a boyfriend."

Still, we spent an hour talking and sharing ideas with each other. And although her saying "no" because she had a boyfriend had nothing to do with my being handicapped, I was pleased she treated me as *"normal."*

For the first time, I came to realize that my disability played a bigger role in my life than I could ever imagine. Before I met Molly, all the challenges in my life weren't that difficult for me to deal with. I was able to get my education and make friends easily, and although I had longed for a relationship ,I hadn't met someone who would inspire me to take a risk until I met Molly.

When I asked her out and she told me she had a boyfriend, even though it wasn't the answer I wanted, I was surprised by how much better I felt after I'd tackled my fear. Sure, you could look at it as a rejection or even bad timing on my part. Still, I had conquered the fear of asking her out. I did it and gained confidence, even though the invitation didn't go my way. In that moment, I really felt empowered and proud of myself that I'd stepped out and taken a chance.

However, the fear that had briefly subsided after I'd asked Molly out returned with a vengeance. The truth is, I couldn't help but feel discouraged and hopeless. Would I *ever* go on a date? Would I *ever* get married?

I kept projecting this fear of rejection onto the rest of my life. Would anybody hire me for a job? Would I find a special woman to marry? As I looked ahead at the life I was headed toward, I felt frozen, petrified like a stone. I could clearly see my life with no future, no one to love, and no career to inspire me. I knew that eventually my friends would get married and have their own families. I started to think of a life as an old man with *no career* and *no family.* That's not a dream; it's a nightmare!

Dramatically afraid for my future, I wanted to give up. But I also knew that if I did, my fate would be sealed—sealed in boredom. Yes, I'm easily bored. And for me, boredom often gives way to daydreaming about the future. As I daydreamed about the life I wanted and in the midst of all my negative energy, I'd hear a little quixotic voice that told me I *could make anything happen*. I recognized that I had all the passion in the world; it was my fear that provoked me into channeling that passion and turning it into motivation.

If you asked me back then if I loved life, I would have said *"no."* But thinking about that time, I realize I'd never loved it more. The fear that I was feeling indicated just how much I *did* love my life and that I cared about my future so much that *I feared for it.*

The fear that I was feeling indicated just how much I did love my life and that I cared about my future so much that I feared for it.

I knew I just had to turn the fear from something *intimidating* to something *motivating*—and I did! My fears urged me to go to the University of Southern California *(USC)*, to become a motivational speaker, and to share my valuable experiences with others.

No matter how confident I am today, a part of me is always scared. Can you imagine a world-class athlete saying to his coach, "I don't need to practice; I'm the best in the world!" Or a CEO saying, "We don't need any marketing because people are going to love us." Andy Grove of Intel was extremely insightful when he said, "Only the paranoid survive."

I'm a highly confident person *and* I believe in what I have to offer, and I fear what the future could bring. Yet as committed lovers have the passion to cope with whatever comes their way,

I have the passion for my own life to deal with whatever comes my way, too.

I understand that failure is always lurking around the corner. I use that fear of failure to my advantage—and so can you.

Don't even aspire to be fearless because being fearless means letting down your guard. Instead, use fear to motivate you.

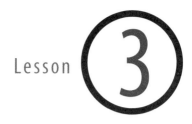

Lesson 3

Make Problem-Solving a Passion

When you're deeply in love with another person, you accept that some things about your loved one will drive you up the wall. You tolerate those things so you can enjoy the relationship. People in good relationships overlook or find a way around each others' shortcomings. After all, you win your love with your personal gifts, not your shortcomings. That's why they don't matter in the long run.

> *You win your love with your personal gifts, not your shortcomings. That's why they don't matter in the long run.*

Many people remark about how I "overcame my disability." I dislike using the word "overcome" because I didn't actually overcome much—I still have physical limitations. The fact is, no matter where I am in life and no matter how successful I become, they will always be there. Barring a medical miracle—something I rarely think about—I will always need help eating, using the restroom, and completing the mundane tasks of daily living.

One of my mentors in the speaking industry told me he started speaking because he was shy and wanted to learn how to relate to people. Today, he boldly speaks to audiences all over the world. So one day, I asked him if he had overcome his shyness. He told me that he still deals with it. For example, before every engagement, he has to call to make sure everything is in place, confirming every last detail about when and where he'll be speaking. He hates making that call; it triggers his shyness. Even though he speaks to thousands of people a night, he still struggles with it. But he knows that to get business, he has to deal with his fears and face them head on.

For me, there's always a sense of uneasiness when I ask a friend to assist me (either using the restroom or helping me eat) because of potential embarrassment. I feel awkward and anxious, but I know ultimately that I *have to* deal with these issues. Any feelings of embarrassment may never go away; it's just the way it is. But I accept the fact that I've got to do what I've got to do to get the help I need—and am always grateful for the help I receive.

What it all boils down to is this: I yearn to make an undesirable situation more desirable. I know that for me to succeed, I need to creatively deal with my limitations and work within the parameters of my situation. In fact, problem-solving like this has become a passion for me.

For example, one semester in junior college, I enrolled in a speech class. Naturally, my first assignment would be to give an informative speech. Not sure of how I was to give my presentation because of my slurred speech, I pulled my professor aside and asked how he wanted me to proceed.

"What do you mean?" he asked, believing I was scared to speak publicly. "You're going to get up there and give your presentation like everyone else."

I quickly responded, "No, no, no. Since I have a speech impediment, shouldn't I use an interpreter?" He said that it was up to me to decide if I needed one. Still, I didn't think I'd convinced him I wasn't afraid of speaking and, more than that, I felt determined to show him I wasn't afraid. I was eager to give a presentation but, practically speaking, I knew I had to get around my speech impediment so others could understand my message. So I devised a skillful way to work with an interpreter and have it heard.

I asked my good friend, Brent, to interpret for me and he agreed. I would say a sentence or two and Brent would repeat what I had just said. This method worked really well. We felt delighted after we saw how well my presentation had been received by the students.

It all boils down to this:
Make an undesirable situation more desirable.

Here's another example. That semester, our professor had described all the attributes of a great speaker, including body movement and hand gestures. Due to my CP, I was lucky if I could keep any parts of my body from moving!

I've always enjoyed telling stories and making people laugh. For me, giving speeches is one way of breaking down walls that my disability creates. It was hard enough just to get a word out, but the answer was getting my points across with the help of my interpreter. In this way, I refused to look at my limitations as setbacks; I regarded them as motivators for creativity. At the end of the semester, I entered a speech contest giving that same presentation about cerebral palsy. I came in third place, feeling ecstatic that I had gotten that far into the process!

From past experiences, I knew that a good way to connect with people was to share stories about my struggles with others. Having the opportunity to do this in front of a class excited me! Today, my disability may keep me from purposeful gesturing and may hinder my ability to effectively show my emotions, but it doesn't stop me from giving speeches. My limitations cause me to focus on delivering great content while using my random, uncontrollable movements with creativity. Here's my motto: Limitations are not stop signs; they're arrows that point people in different directions.

Limitations are not stop signs; they're arrows that point people in different directions.

Be mindful of the difference between a legitimate limitation and a self-imposed one. Let me explain what I mean.

Before the beginning of the semester, I actually tried to get this particular speech class waived. I told myself there was *no way* I could give a presentation. To my benefit, I failed in getting it waived, which made me focus on dealing with my disability instead of using it as an excuse. Indeed, that one class made me realize that I loved speaking. I loved it so much, I made it my career!

Of course, realism plays a role that can't be ignored. I can't be like my mentor Frank Miles who juggles fire on a unicycle at the end of his keynote addresses. No matter what, I will never be able to do that, and my audiences are lucky that I won't attempt to do so! It's not one of my talents, nor is it one of my goals.

On the other side of the coin, underestimating possibilities can play a role, too, like I did when I wanted to waive my speech class. Never underestimate what you can do. And, just as important, don't overestimate your abilities either. The solution for me is to focus on what I *can* do—that is, convey to my audiences the lessons I've learned for success in the face of daunting odds.

Never underestimate what you can do.
And, just as important, don't
overestimate your abilities either.

In a love relationship, limitations are similar to traits that may irritate you about another person. But you can always find ways to deal with them to enjoy the relationship, don't you?

I believe you must also do this when loving your own life. **You cannot simply love only the good parts!** Okay, you may never love the bad, but you still have to deal with unsavory or unpleasant happenings. You'll find that how you deal with them in the moment affects your happiness and success every day.

I am sure there are parts of your day that you can't stand, such as taking out the trash, pumping gas, or sitting in rush hour traffic. To accomplish your goals, you know that you have to put up with these less-than-desirable aspects of life. Just like in a relationship, there will be times where your mate is sick, or is running late, or is just being flat-out boring. But you understand that to build a loving relationship with someone, the illusion of always having a wonderful time dissolves pretty quickly. The way I see it, you have to accept the unpleasant or boring parts because you relish the payoff.

Similarly, if you fall in love with life, those annoying tasks like pumping gas or sitting in traffic won't seem so bad because of the overall benefit you get. You simply declare, "I'm putting up with this for the greater good of being fulfilled in a key relationship. There's no true love that doesn't include the bad parts."

Start today dealing with your own annoying limitations in a positive, creative manner, and let them point you in the direction of your success!

You cannot simply love only the good parts of life!

Lesson 4

Don't Limit Your Thinking

You wouldn't walk up to someone you're romantically interested in at a party and say, "Hey, you don't want to dance with me." That's a big "no-no." From time to time, life will say "no" to you, but you don't ever want to start the conversation by saying "no" to life.

One of the most dangerous limitations you might face is your own thinking. Here's an example from my life. Growing up, I never had anybody except my parents help me in the restroom, so I always assumed that I would have to go to a college that was within driving distance of my parents' house. I thought there was *no way* another person would help me in the restroom. I also thought I'd find it too humiliating to ask anyone else to help—not to mention that I doubted anyone would want to assist me. This type of thinking prevented me from believing I could ever go away to college. I had convinced myself that living away from home was 100% out of the question.

One day, Dr. Jerry Fecht, my professor at Moorpark

Community College, suggested I move out of my parents' house and go away to a university. I said I didn't think I'd ever be able to attend a four-year school that was more than half an hour away because I required so much help. He told me point blank I could do it—like it was *that* easy.

I'd say Jerry is definitely in love with his life. In every lecture that I heard Jerry give, he talked about romance and love. I could see the excitement in his face and hear it in his voice. He loved making the students laugh. As a professor, he always taught his students to go as far as they could go.

When I took his class at one of the hardest times of my life, I couldn't help but feel uplifted every time I walked out. But I assumed that, being disabled, different rules applied to me. Jerry knew I was a good student and his suggestion to "go for it" flattered me, but I thought that he didn't understand my circumstances. When I pointed them out, he simply said, "Get help." I rolled my eyes at that one. "Yeah, right," I protested. "Jerry doesn't understand the intricacies of my life. He doesn't know how I get ready in the morning, or how I have to get through my daily routines."

Instead of completely dismissing his idea, though, I started thinking about what he said, even picking the college I wanted in an area outside of my safe zone. Four days after he said "go for it," I made a tentative decision. I'd move out of my parents' house some day so I could go to a university. I even picked one—the University of Southern California—because of its high academic standards and because a close friend of mine loved it so much. At this point, I had no idea how I'd do it.

My self-imposed limitations had prevented me from thinking big before, but that day, I knew I had to try. I had no road map, but my passionate desire to have a bona fide university life guided me forward.

I knew I'd face many setbacks, but I persisted and I got accepted at USC. What compelled me? Two things: Envy of my friend Arie, who you'll meet in Lesson Five. And my decision not to let limited thinking prevent me from pursuing my dream.

I honestly had no idea whether moving away from home was a stupid notion or a realistic goal. Still, I wanted to make it happen. Yes, I'd have to work extra hard and get assistance from many people, but my gut said it would be worth every effort.

Over the course of two years, I had to hire more than ten people in order for me to live on campus and graduate from USC. My assistants did everything from organize my notes to help me get ready in the morning. On a typical morning, one of my assistants would help me shower and dress and feed me breakfast. Throughout the day, various students would help me with my class work, including typing papers, taking tests, and doing take-home assignments. Even reading required help; because of my lack of head control, it's difficult for me to focus on the pages at all times. Then someone would assist me at the end of the day, cleaning up, brushing my teeth, and getting me ready for bed.

Getting through the course work and all the degree requirements challenged me, but I loved the effort, knowing it was well worth it! I made it through and accepted a degree in marketing from the Marshall School of Business at USC in the spring of 2001.

In the midst of this accomplishment, though, somehow I knew my life lessons had barely begun. Here's an example.

In my last year at USC, I attended a career fair. Like every other senior, I dressed up in a suit and tie and armed myself with business cards and copies of my resume for networking. The day after the fair, I got a phone call at my campus apartment from a company representative who wanted to talk about a job. Needless to say, I was excited. When I talked to the HR director on the phone, he asked me to come in for an interview.

I learned that this company wanted a salesperson who could drive around. I can't drive and due to my speech impediment, I assumed I'd never be an effective salesperson. Who would pay me for that? So instead of going to the interview, I politely told the HR director, "I'm sorry. I'm the wrong guy for this job."

The worst thing that could happen is not getting a "no"; it's not trying for it at all.

Even years later, I regret saying that because it showed how I'd limited the possibilities in my life. I could have hired somebody to drive me around and facilitate a conversation between myself and clients. Limited thinking gets me nowhere.

At the time, I was 23 and naïve. I only bring up this story to illustrate a poignant lesson I'm passing on to you. I have no idea if the hiring manager of that company would seriously consider me as a candidate, but it doesn't matter. I remind myself of that story to push myself even further to succeed.

I also remind myself that it's not up to me to make decisions for others. If you see a job opening and think you're not qualified, don't automatically assume you'd never get hired. Let your potential employer make that decision! The worst thing that could happen is not getting a "no"; it's not trying for it at all.

In the past, I had made decisions on behalf of my friends, such as deciding I could never travel with them because it would be too much for them to assist me with intimate tasks. That's just like deciding I wasn't the right candidate for the sales job.

Today, I look back and realize that decisions like these don't belong to me. They belong to the people who might take a chance on me!

What are you deciding on behalf of others?
And what about the people you won't
let take a chance on you?

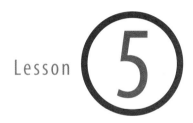

Use Envy to Ignite Your Passion

Telling and listening to stories have always been part of our culture. At one time or another, we thoroughly enjoyed hearing a good love story. Why? It's about more than getting caught up in the story. We're waking up the romantic side in us. More than that, we envy the love being shown between the main characters.

A well-portrayed love story brings out desires of being touched, warmed, and uplifted. These same emotions motivate us to find or create a love like the one we've just observed. I consider that a form of envy.

To me, the meaning of envy differs from jealousy. Jealousy assumes that if you don't have something another person has, that person shouldn't have it either. On the flip side, when you are envious, you aspire to be in a similar position as someone whose life you admire. Have you noticed that successful people love talking about what they do? They love exchanging information because it makes them feel secure and confident. In many cases, they're simply looking for ears to hear about how successful they are and how they got there.

In Lesson One, I encouraged you to imagine and visualize the life you want to ignite your passion. One way of igniting that passion is becoming envious of people who have been successful in achieving what you want to do. Actively seek and emulate people whose careers and/or lives you admire.

Becoming envious of people who have been successful in achieving what you want to do can ignite your own passion.

Here's how envy sparked my desires to get my degree at USC.

In the fall of 1997 when I was starting an accounting class at Moorpark Community College, I noticed a young man sitting in the desk in front of me. Dressed in business attire, Arie Paller looked professional and grown up. I figured he had to be at least 25 or 26, but in actuality, he was only 17. Arie was making plans to move on to the University of Southern California as soon as he fulfilled his general requirements at this community college. We instantly hit it off and during the following semester, he quickly became one of my closest friends. Over the years, we've developed a close, lasting friendship.

I was fascinated listening to Arie's experiences, and as I got to know him better, I recognized a bit of myself in him. He proved to be everything I believe I *would have been* had I not been born with a disability. Arie was a hard worker, disciplined, and accomplished. If he saw something he wanted, he'd go after it until he got it. Although we had similar goals in life, Arie was well on his way to achieving his goals. Attending

USC promised him a bright future.

At that time, Arie's life clearly loved him a lot but it felt like my life didn't love me at all. Sure, I could say I had all the passion in the world, but I figured that life was for able-bodied people, not someone like me who could barely take care of himself. Deep down, I felt like a lonely heart reading a novel about someone else's romance!

So what did I do? I used the emotion of envy to ignite the passion necessary for me to reach for my true potential.

As I mentioned before, this time in my life was particularly hard. I didn't know if I'd ever land a job; I didn't know if I'd ever find a girlfriend. As a result, I started living vicariously through Arie. At the time, he was heading toward the type of life that I thought belonged to me. Through his experiences, my own vision came to light. I saw what my life would be like if I were not handicapped.

At the same time, I felt compelled to communicate to him how lucky he was to be in a position to take advantage of every opportunity. As a friend, I was happy for him and always looked forward to hearing about more of his experiences. As much as it hurt me, I wanted *him* to succeed—and I wanted to be his cheerleader.

My envy grew, but at the same time, a little voice in my head got louder and louder. It said, "Sourena, you have a chance as well."

I took this opportunity to gravitate more toward Arie. I wanted to know what it was like to move out and go off to a university. Not only was Arie planning that, but he went off to Europe on a vacation and had an incredible time. At that time,

I thought I could never go on a vacation without my parents—not even a simple road trip with my friends, much less go on a fabulous trip to a foreign country.

Shortly after returning from Europe, Arie started classes at USC and called me to tell me what amazing experiences he was enjoying. Again I told him how fortunate I thought he was and eagerly listened to all the details. He talked about his dorm room, his cool roommate, and how liberating it felt to be away from home. I felt happy for him, yet hearing about how great everything was for him frustrated me, too.

That phone call turned out to be a pivotal moment in my life. The evening he called, my parents were entertaining guests in the living room so I took Arie's phone call in another part of the house. After talking with him, I didn't even want to return to being with our guests; I just wanted to be left alone. It broke my heart hearing about a lifestyle I so desperately wanted. My parents tried to coax me to come out and visit, but I turned them down. Our conversation weighed heavy on my mind.

After that, I began crying. The tears and lamentations came billowing out: It was unfair that Arie could have this amazing life and chase his dreams, and I couldn't. Nothing against him, mind you; *I just wanted that, too.*

I thought about all the reasons I couldn't do what he was doing: USC is too far from home, my parents wouldn't be around to help me, I'd face a myriad of unknown complications that going away would present, and on and on. When I thought about the reasons that I should pursue going to a university, I could only come up with one: I wanted to.

My dad saw how upset I was and tried to console me. And I don't know exactly what happened next except that I just blurted out, "I want to go to USC."

Immediately, I couldn't believe I'd said that, yet doing it energized me. Saying the words out loud to someone else made it more of a possibility for me. I wanted a life like Arie's so badly that I decided to start taking action, even if it only took the form of making a powerful statement to my dad. It felt so good to say it, to put my heart on the line like that.

And while I knew it wouldn't be easy, going to USC just felt right. Even though I'd wanted to make this decision after Dr. Fecht put the idea into my head, the envy I felt suddenly kicked my motivation into high gear.

A year later, I started taking classes at the University of Southern California. I had hoped Arie would help me get acclimated to life away from home. We'd even talked about rooming together for my first year, but that's when Arie got accepted into the university's Semester Abroad program. While I was extremely excited for him and all the wonderful adventures he'd have overseas, it made my transition to life away on campus that much tougher. Because I didn't have Arie to lean on, I also had to deal with feeling uncomfortable. Although the idea of making new friends and finding my way around campus seemed daunting, they turned out to be character-building experiences for me. I could never truly measure the sense of independence and pride I'd gained by the end of that first semester.

When Arie came back to campus for the second semester, we shared two classes and spent a lot of time together working on group projects. And on most Thursday nights, he'd have me over to his apartment for dinner—some of the best times I'd had at USC. Best of all, every time I saw Arie on campus, I got an incredible reminder that my life was loving me back.

Arie and I have remained close friends over the years. I've watched him live out life experiences such as dating, living abroad, and embarking on successful business ventures. I understand that it takes more effort and time for me to accomplish my goals than for others. Still, I continue to use my envy of his success to inspire me and push me harder.

As I look back, I see that I'd become excited about Arie's experiences and I let myself fantasize about living them. I envied his life so much that it drove me to find a way to live a life that satisfied me!

Envy got me out of my shell—and it could motivate you, too.

How do you really know what you want? I suggest you keep your eyes open and observe the people around you, always looking to identify what others are doing and determining what changes you might want to make. Then mirror the actions of people you admire.

As an example, I enjoy networking with highly successful entrepreneurs and speakers, asking them specific questions about their careers. I love hearing where they're going and where they've been. I listen to their experiences and even imagine myself in their positions. They understand that I'm eager to do "whatever it takes" to attain positions similar to theirs. They *inspire* me.

It's important to not lose your own identity in the process of getting to know successful people. Even though you might emulate people you admire, make the effort to tailor the expectations and lessons in this book to your own gifts and limitations.

> *It's important not to lose your own identity in the process of getting to know successful people.*

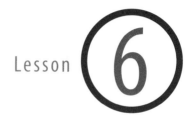

Lesson 6

Let Need Fuel Your Success

W hen lovers say, "I need you," they mean, "I need you to make my life complete." They don't mean, "I'd like to have you in my life, but I guess I'll live if I don't."

I like to visualize this idea in the form of a spectrum. On one end, you have a "want"; on the other end, you have an absolute "need." One hundred percent of the time, you aim to satisfy your needs before your wants. For instance, if you want a really cool shirt that's on sale for $20 but you need to get gas because your car is running on empty, you'll satisfy your need before your want. Well, either that or walk to the store to buy that shirt!

The Rolling Stones wrote:

You can't always get what you want
But if you try sometimes,
You might find you get what you need.

These lyrics convey that needs can be extremely powerful motivators capable of evoking passion and dedication.

I believe that the more you feel you need success, the more likely you are to achieve it. For example, you've probably had times when you were financially strapped for cash and suddenly the car broke down, or you had to pay an unexpected medical bill, or your kids simply needed uniforms for Little League baseball. You scrounged and saved, and finally found a way to fulfill that need.

Do you see that having needs increases the passion necessary to fuel your success?

> *Having needs increases the passion*
> *necessary to fuel your success.*

In my situation, I realize I have no safety net, which means that I can't get an ordinary job as easily as others can. If I don't succeed in meeting my goals, I could end up in a group home for the disabled with nothing to do for a job. Imagining that fate makes me desperate for success. It's that desperation—that need—that drives me every day.

To be specific, I need to be able to provide for a family of my own. I need to give back to society everything it has afforded me. And I need to somehow repay all the people who have helped me along the way. These are all good things. Why? Because we're driven to satisfy our needs before we satisfy our wants.

Most people survive on what money they make and don't feel compelled to become financially successful. For some people, financial success is a "want" that's regarded as a convenience that makes their lives easier.

But for me, financial success is a "need"—a full-blown necessity. You see, I need a handicap-accessible van to transport me to all my business appointments. Although the van cost about as much as a brand new Mercedes Benz, I had to buy it because I needed it. And if you really needed a Mercedes the way I need my van, you'd have one in your garage right now. (I better not get any e-mails from angry spouses saying that I said you *"need"* a Mercedes Benz!)

Highly successful people have the hunger to go after what they believe they need. They're driven not only by their wants, but by their absolute need to go further, to push themselves to the limit and beyond. I suggest that you don't be afraid to let yourself need things.

What do you consider a *"need"* versus a *"want"* in your life?

Don't be afraid to let yourself need things. Need is an extremely powerful motivator capable of evoking passion and dedication.

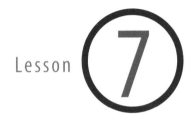

Lesson 7

Keep the Change

Perhaps two people in a relationship really love one another and have for a long time. Yet something doesn't feel right. They crave direction to make a change. Their relationship has to evolve—for better or for worse. Whatever happens, they'll always face change.

In case you haven't noticed, the days of getting a job and keeping it until retirement are over. Every other day, an insight or innovation changes our careers and our chosen industries, which means we must be flexible and willing to adapt to those changes.

Sometimes finding out we're wrong about our choices in life (like finding out you can't get anywhere on your initial career path) can be the best thing that happens. For example, I was wrong when I thought I could never go to a university away from home. In that case, being wrong put me on a better path and I'm grateful for that.

One of my mentors, Dr. Terry Paulson, uses this great line: *"People crave a direction, even if it's wrong."* Here's an example of this principle.

When I applied to community college, one of the counselors who worked in the Office for Disabled Students helped me pick out my classes for the first semester. She suggested I only take three classes instead of five because of my disability. Although I was uncomfortable with the set up, I agreed to it. Unfortunately, this agreement set me back big time; instead of taking two years to complete an associate's degree program, it took me four years.

I regret that I didn't reevaluate my situation during those four years while following the direction that the counselor gave me. I had convinced myself that I was plugging away unbothered by the set up—until the end of my third year. At that time, I knew I could be achieving more, much more, in that environment! So in the next two semesters, I took more classes and pushed myself harder than ever.

Up to that point, I had relied on my mom to help me with my schoolwork. I realized that if I wanted to reach my full potential, I would have to hire students to assist me because my mom was working 40 hours a week and couldn't help me if I wanted to be a full-time student.

The next semester, I upped my course load again. Needless to say, many aspects of doing that proved uncomfortable, especially because I was challenged to take on the extra work as well as doing it without my mom's constant help. At first, it was extremely difficult to find outside help. On campus, I just asked for assistance from random strangers, other students, professors, anybody who came by. This embarrassed me at times, as I've mentioned before, but by the time I figured out how to find assistants, I had become so independent that my grades were better in my classes that semester than the ones I took earlier. Once I hired people to help me, I was so used to doing so many things for myself that I'd call on my assistants as needed but I never leaned on them as a crutch because of laziness.

The worst part of taking a small class load was not knowing that I even needed to change my mindset. When I realized how necessary that had become, I figured out a different path. Changing proved to be uncomfortable at first, but I learned to embrace it and love it. It's easy to get used to certain ways of doing things. That's why it's critical to have the foresight to know when change is necessary, even though making the change feels uncomfortable (and it almost always does). It's a lot easier to put up with a familiar scenario than smash through that comfort zone and learn from it.

I suggest that if something isn't working the way you want, you try something else. Did you know that insanity is doing something over and over the same way and expecting different results?

It's critical to have the foresight to know when change is necessary, even though making the change feels uncomfortable.

Straight out of college, I wanted to get into advertising or public relations and tried my best to break through and find a job in those fields. I e-mailed companies, I went to networking events, I offered to do an internship for no pay. I became acquainted with a few companies that I would have given my right arm to work for! (Well, that's not a good analogy because I can't do anything with my right arm, but you know what I mean.)

Yet sometimes the answer really is "no." When I was looking for a job, I usually went alone, which created questions in the prospective employers' minds, partly because they had a hard time understanding my speech. I tried to convey to them that as soon as I got a job, I would hire an assistant to work with me. Later, when I started hiring people for my own speaking business, I discovered that every time I interviewed somebody, I would question how this person might work and what could go wrong. I can only imagine what thoughts went through any prospective employer's mind while interviewing me!

The most difficult part of the job hunt was knowing that, given the right chance, I could excel. I actually came close to landing a PR job when a recruiter from Fox Studios invited me to interview in a big conference room on the lot of Fox studios. Beforehand, I had researched the company relentlessly and thought I interviewed for it well, but the job never came to fruition.

That's when I realized that landing a job wasn't my goal; rather, it was *creating a career* that inspired me. So I started networking with professional speakers through the National Speakers Association and found my calling. When I was networking in the PR industry, I felt like an outsider begging to get in. I rarely received constructive feedback on what I was doing, right or wrong. When I started networking in the speaking industry, other speakers gave me valuable advice, like helping me figure out ways to deliver my speech and giving me feedback on its content.

If your goal is to create a career that inspires you, then what has to change in your life?

As soon as I started meeting speakers, I instantly developed close relationships and I knew my career could move forward because of their support. I've faced dozens of challenges and setbacks, but not enough to deter me from this career path. Among the speakers I've been meeting, I feel as though I belong.

As I learned more about the speaking industry, I realized that the things I wanted to do—designing press kits, collaborating on website designs, creating and implementing marketing plans—were needed activities within my reach as a speaker running my own business.

In addition, I realized that I could travel for business, which had seemed so impossible before. As a speaker, not only do I get to travel, but I also have the opportunity to inspire people for whom travel looms as a barrier.

Yes, I'd found my professional home among professional speakers who seem more innovative, flexible, and willing to think outside the box than the world of mainstream, corporate America—especially when it comes to someone with a disability. I'm not slamming corporate America; rather, I'm emphasizing that while I was desperately trying to fit into that world, it wasn't until I made a drastic change in my career path that I was truly able to find my calling.

My goal had always been to get into the business world. By starting my own business, I was able to accomplish that without corporate America. Who needs more advertising, anyway?

The same could be true for you. Check in with your intuition and don't be afraid to change your path.

Check in with your intuition and don't be afraid to change your path.

A need to keep changing applies to relationships, too. The person you marry when you're in your 20s changes a lot over the next few decades, guaranteed. To keep the passion in their relationship alive, a couple can't be rigid with each other and with the way they live their lives. And being flexible enough to handle any bumps on the road makes the journey more fun!

In the world of relationships, perhaps you can relate to a time when you had a crush on an attractive member of the opposite sex—an attraction that was never reciprocated. No matter how hard you tried, you had to determine it would never work out.

I, too, experienced that when I met a young woman named Hannah—a pretty brunette with curly hair. We talked the whole evening and our conversation flowed so well, it seemed that she was having a good time talking with me. I got her contact information and we started e-mailing each other. We even had coffee together a couple of times. Every time I asked her to go out via e-mail, I would impatiently wait at the computer for her response. I assumed that if I wanted something to happen, it was up to me entirely. I soon realized, however, that no matter how hard I tried, forming a relationship with Hannah just wasn't happening. After all, the world doesn't revolve around any one of us. While I really liked her, I started realizing that trying too hard for a relationship with her was not going to get me the results that I wanted.

Both people in a relationship can easily fall into a routine, letting the romance and initial attraction die down or even die out. To avoid this, it's important to know when change is necessary and constantly reinvent the relationship.

Having the passion to live your dreams may mean tweaking what you're doing or even taking new paths. But if you're alert and willing to change, I believe the path that allows you to contribute the most will open up to you—in a way that allows you to love your life more fully.

The path that allows you to contribute the most will open up to you—in a way that allows you to love your life more fully.

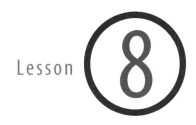

Take Advantage of Luck

When you meet the love of your life, it feels like luck. You talk about how lucky you are and how you hope the passion and the bliss of it all will never wear off.

So if you want your relationship to stay passionate, do what it takes to make sure you keep it that way! Too many people think that their effort is complete once they've found their *"true love."* Don't be fooled. It's constant work to maintain a great relationship with a special person. You'll pay a huge price if you neglect or take for granted such a great gift.

Luck has played a huge part in my life. Growing up, I was lucky to have loving parents who help me with what I need every day. They've always been there when I needed them, and when I don't need them, they let me live my own life. What good fortune to have such wonderful parents!

Other aspects of my life have been well speckled with both luck and learning. For example, in 2002, I excitedly attended my first job networking event. I introduced myself to people, gave them my resume, and collected business cards. When I came home, I threw the business cards into a box. I thought that was the end of my part in this.

But nothing happened.

I had to learn quickly. I realized that if I wanted a job, I couldn't wait by the phone and expect an employer to randomly call and ask me, "Do you need a job?" *I* was the one who had the need, therefore *I* was the one who'd have to convince decision-makers that *I* belonged in their company. And especially because of my unique circumstances, I needed to be aggressive about communicating that.

Early in 2006, I visited the Los Angeles Chapter of the National Speakers Association. I wanted to attend this event primarily to network within the industry. The program topic, *"How to Get Media Exposure,"* featured a raffle for the opportunity to pitch story ideas to those members of the media in attendance that day. Eight winners out of 100 attendees were named—and I was one of them. You can definitely call that luck, but as soon as I won, my assistant and I had to come up with a compelling speech.

Luck is the product of taking advantage of opportunities presented to you.

When we got back to my office, we turned the interest generated at the event into something tangible—a press release, which we wrote and sent out to select media outlets. A reporter contacted me and, a few weeks later, I was featured in the *Los Angeles Business Journal.* Then two weeks after the article came out, I got a phone call from a producer at the local NBC TV affiliate. They asked if they could do a profile about my speaking business as well as allow the TV crew to film my speech. As a result, I spent countless hours preparing a seminar, which I conducted for an audience in front of the cameras. Shortly after, a feature story about me aired four times in four days on KNBC Channel 4 News in Los Angeles.

All this happened because I used hard work to turn luck into something that could help me and my business. Do you see that luck is not purely the product of random things happening to you? It comes from taking advantage of opportunities presented to you.

Similarly, to find a mate, you can't sit home and do nothing. Be proactive. These days, with Internet dating becoming more and more prominent, you can even be proactive without ever leaving your home! The point is, you have to put forth effort to attract the mate you want. It's like playing the lottery. The saying, "You can't win if you don't play" is a worn cliché that continues to be true. Even though the odds for your winning the lottery are minuscule at best, one fact prevails: Every single winning lottery ticket has come as the result of a proactive measure taken. Whether it's a group's weekly purchase or simply an extra buck spent on a single ticket at your local convenience store, that action was rewarded with a winning ticket. Translated, that means even if the "perfect" mate sits next to you at a club, you still have to say hello.

There are certainly aspects of life that seem to randomly happen by chance. But today's "chance encounter" becomes tomorrow's story of "love at first sight." You have to be prepared to take advantage of luck when it presents itself to you. It may take major effort on your part, or it may be as simple as buying one lottery ticket, but when you nurture an optimistic and hopeful heart, you can maximize that luck and often create your own.

When you nurture an optimistic and hopeful heart, you can maximize the luck that comes your way and often create your own.

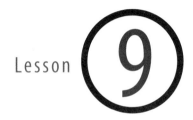

Lesson 9

Trust Your Instinct

Is there such a book called *Love Your Mate and He/She Will Love You Back?* And if there is, what advice could it give so your mate would always love you back!

Let's face it. We'll never have all the information necessary to make our mate constantly happy, therefore we must largely rely on a vital force called instinct.

Business schools teach strategies under ideal conditions. When I graduated and started my own business, I discovered that real conditions are anything but ideal! To maximize your potential under non-ideal conditions (or *"life"* as it is called), it's wise to trust your instincts.

Now, I'm not suggesting your instincts are always right. You still need concrete information to make concrete decisions. But most of the time, you simply won't have all of the information you think you need to make a decision. That's when you examine information but also rely on your instinct to move forward.

Here's an example. In the middle of 2004, which was three years after I graduated from USC, I played with the idea of going back to the university and earning my master's degree in communications. I hesitated to go, but I investigated the possibility anyway. I had been working out of my house for three years and missed daily interactions with people. Luckily, I met the director of a nonprofit organization and convinced him to give me a full scholarship to USC, including books, tuition, and living expenses. (When I attended USC as an undergrad, I didn't know that I had a chance at government funds that would help me pay for my assistants).

I remembered brimming with excitement when I first went to USC in the fall of 1999. I couldn't wait for this new challenge to begin. At the time, I kept wondering if this might be a mistake. Riddled with doubt mixed in with anticipation, I didn't know if I could make it on my own at the university. I could have gone to two schools closer to my house that would have cost me nothing and allowed me to rely on my parents for help with whatever I needed. But despite these thoughts and feelings, I couldn't stop the momentum. My instinct told me to enroll at USC.

As mentioned earlier, the most compelling reason to go to USC was that it *felt right*. Of course, that's not what I told my family. I said that the education was better, and that I could make connections there I couldn't make at the schools nearby. I didn't know if these arguments were true, but they sounded reasonable at the time. How often do we apply reason to justify our gut feelings?

When I applied to attend grad school, however, it just didn't feel right, even though I kept saying, "How could I go wrong? This time, I have a full scholarship and funds for my assistants." So I took one class in 2005 to get my feet wet and loved being back in an academic setting.

Then a few weeks into the first semester, I attended a convention for the National Speakers Association where I was surrounded by 400 professional speakers. Most of them had made successful careers out of speaking and that made an impression on me. I told myself that was where I belonged. Two days after the convention, I withdrew from my university class, deciding that my focus needed to be on my speaking business. I honestly couldn't see how grad school would advance my objective of becoming a professional speaker.

Life is a series of decisions. No matter how much information you gather, you still face unknowns, which is why I encourage you to mix rational decision-making with your instincts. When you do, you'll choose what's right for you in the long run.

When you mix rational decision-making with your instincts, you'll choose what's right for you in the long run.

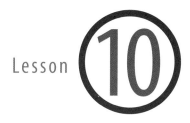

Be Open to New Experiences

A wise man once said, "If you don't take any risks, then nothing bad or good will ever happen to you."

Do you know people who are so afraid of getting hurt that they can't let themselves romantically fall in love? It reminds me of the famous quotation about loving and losing. Take a look at the full stanza:

I hold it true, whate'er befall;
I feel it, when I sorrow most;
'Tis better to have loved and lost
Than never to have loved at all.

Alfred Lord Tennyson wrote these lines in 1850 about the loss of a dear friend in his poem titled *"In Memoriam."* To paraphrase, when the poet feels most sad about the death of his beloved friend, he still knows it's better to have experienced the love, despite the pain.

In this Lesson, I'm simply asking you to apply this idea more widely to all of life, knowing that "'Tis better to have lived and lost than never to have lived at all."

Inevitably, you'll fall on your rear end from time to time. Just remember it's the price you pay for a life worth living—and I think you'll find it easy enough to accept.

I also live my life that way. I am emotional about every single aspect of it. I want to win, and I don't want to lose. Much of the time, I feel like I'm riding an emotional roller coaster. For me and for most people, the bigger the roller coaster, the greater the risk—and the more possibilities open up.

I also pay attention to "the bigger the climb, the bigger the fall" credo. The reason some people don't like to ride big roller coasters is that they don't want to experience the fall. But to succeed in life in the way you want to live it, you need to ride bigger and scarier roller coasters—and the more emotional you feel, the better!

To be emotionally present in your life, you need to love winning and hate losing.

Here's another example. When your favorite sports team finds itself on a winning streak, it's tough to see your heroes lose. You're so frustrated when they do, you can't sleep. You call and complain to everybody who might remotely care, saying, "Can you believe those guys lost?" But when your team gets stuck in a losing streak and lose yet another game, you say,

"Oh, well." You don't call your friends and you don't lose any sleep. You simply don't care as much.

The game of life commands you to be emotionally involved with your "team" every day, whether you're having a winning streak or not. It doesn't care if you're having a good day or a bad day. It doesn't care if times don't get better or couldn't get worse. To be emotionally present in your life, you need to love winning and hate losing.

When I have a good day, I go to bed with a big old smile on my face. I'm eager to wake up the next morning and smile all over again. When I have a bad day, I can't wait to have a better day!

A few months before I decided to go to USC, I struggled with the fact that I might live my whole life without getting to live out my dreams. I wanted to give up. I was tired of being in a rut. I tried to convince myself that I should give up on every single one of my dreams. I didn't think my dreams even suited me!

In addition, I thought dreams were only for people who had the ability to walk, talk, and take care of themselves. They weren't for me. Perhaps I was trying to become numb to the pain, to become inured. But, something inside me said "No!"

A couple of times, I freaked out. I thought that I'd miss achieving success by a mile. People around me worried that my heavy emotional mood was hurting me. But in reality, I was getting ready for the future.

Once I reached the age of twenty, I was becoming more and more aware of how much it hurt not to go after my goals.

I knew I couldn't keep living my life the same way year after year. I despised where I was heading. I couldn't wait to get back on a meaningful track. And the minute I decided to go to USC, I took control. I decided to love my life absolutely!

I suggest that, to live your dreams, you must accept the fact that you'll experience difficult days. The antidote? Having a strong enough passion that gets you through anything life throws at you. I contend it's more important to be in love with your life when nothing is going right than when everything looks rosy. Don't get used to a bad situation; let it get under your skin. That way, you're more likely to make a change.

Don't get used to a bad situation; let it get under your skin. That way, you're more likely to make a change.

When you're riding at the bottom of that roller coaster, know that you'll start to climb higher and higher. Soon, you'll be at the top of the world.

Concluding Lesson

A s you know, in any worthwhile love relationship, you'll experience good days and bad. So it goes with the pursuit of success. No one said success would be easy or copasetic all of the time!

It begins, though, with a flexible dream and a promise to yourself that you'll do anything to chase that dream, no matter the obstacles. You have to be willing to use every single one of your resources. If you notice something missing, then you have two choices: to either find it or make what you've got work better.

Let me repeat a core message of mine stated in Lesson One: *Limitations are not excuses, but arrows to help point you in the right direction.* I live this message every day. I know I can't give a keynote address totally on my own, so I have an interpreter to assist me. I can't walk up the stairs, but I can use an elevator. My motto: *Work with what you have instead of lamenting about what you don't have.*

Isn't it ironic that a guy like me with a severe speech impediment can find a way to become a professional speaker? That proves that more possibilities exist than you can ever imagine!

Don't be limited by your own thinking. There is a *fabulous* life waiting for you; go out and grab it. It will take a lot of work, but if you are motivated, doors will open for you.

> ## *There is a fabulous life waiting for you; go out and grab it.*

I can honestly say that I am motivated 100% of the time. Being motivated doesn't mean that I don't get discouraged or I never have a bad day. Being motivated means that I'm always on the quest to make my life better.

For many, staying motivated is an everyday struggle. I'm fortunate, however, to have phenomenal friends and great mentors. They give a piece of their lives to me so that my life becomes better. I'm privileged to experience the gift of loving life on a daily basis. Because of it, I enjoy each and every moment I'm able to share with the incredible people around me. Their presence alone inspires me to succeed. I would love to name them all, but there are just too many—which, I guess, makes me a very fortunate man.

Although I've experienced times when I thought I had to give up on my life's dreams, I never stopped loving life. And I never will. Because I stay motivated, I look forward to the future enthusiastically. That helps me enjoy each present moment, no matter how good, bad, or just plain difficult it may be.

Let me be crystal clear on this. Loving life means having the passion to go after your dreams; it doesn't mean you should always be happy or accepting of everything that happens to you. No day goes by when my disability doesn't inconvenience or frustrate me, but I roll on. I do so because I love myself enough to know that by taking a chance on tomorrow, I give myself a chance at the success and happiness I desire.

The minute I start blaming my problems on my disability, I lose control over my life. The minute I accept that my life *is* my responsibility, I get empowered.

I'm no saint. I have moments every day when I blame my problems on my disability. I constantly struggle to break out of that mindset. Some days are easier than others. The only constant is my love of life.

I was recently asked this question by a reporter: "How do you know when you've made it?" Without skipping a beat, I responded, "When I'm sitting on a couch with my wife in my own house." I'm in love with that dream for my life; I'm determined to make that happen. Being successful, buying a home, starting a family. I'm in love with that dream so much that the thought of not having it or achieving it scares me to death.

When you love another person enough, your heart tells you not to give up on him or her, so relentlessly you pursue your desires. You love that person unconditionally. You love him or her regardless of whether you receive love in return. You press on with the faith and hope that one day, you will be loved in return. As the song "Nature Boy" written by Eden Ahbez states: *"The greatest thing you'll ever learn is just to love and be loved in return."*

In love affairs, you may relentlessly love someone only to be let down by that person in the end. But if you love your life, your dreams, and your unending pursuit of success, then you cannot fail!

If you love yourself and your dreams—
flaws and all—your life will have
no choice but to reciprocate!

It may sound corny, but I've realized that the best reward of loving my life is that I get to help people live out their dreams.

Please take a moment right now to put down this book and take a long look inside you. In this quiet, open space within, contemplate this thought: Whoever you are, whatever limitations you have, however lofty your dreams, know that you are now closer to achieving those dreams!

Just by reading these Ten Lessons, you have already begun taking better control of your life. You have loved yourself enough to dedicate the time to reading this book. And now you have the lessons to continue falling in love with your life!

I assure you that this book is not a bunch of clichés—this book is my life filled with concepts on how I do more than *"just get by."*

What is success for me? It's a never-ending journey that includes having a large network, being accomplished in my profession, helping others build their dreams, and enjoying myself while doing so. To ensure all this happens, I love my life every day!

You can accomplish your dreams as well; you'll see. Love your life and it will love you back.

About the Author

Sourena Vasseghi is a man of exceptional accomplishments. A successful businessman and keynote speaker, Sourena lives life to the fullest despite his severe case of cerebral palsy.

Although he is wheelchair-bound, has a prominent speech impediment, and needs assistance in most of his daily activities, he has always refused to let his disabilities stand in his way. At an early age, determined to fulfill his social as well as intellectual potential, he moved from special education classes to a mainstream academic setting. He went on to earn a bachelor of science in business administration with an emphasis in marketing from the University of Southern California *(USC)*. Graduation ceremonies at USC in 2001 garnered him a standing ovation from the faculty and hundreds of fellow students and their families.

Sourena believes that although life is challenging, each of us bears the responsibility of making things happen for ourselves. In *Love Your Life and It Will Love You Back*, he shares the principles that have been essential to his success and positive outlook. His ten life lessons inspire his readers with a renewed passion for love, life, and achievement.